Copyright © 2024 Barry Pena

All rights reserved. No part of this publication may be reproduced or distributed in any form or by any means, or stored in a database or retrieval system, without the prior written permission of the author, except where permitted by law.

Legal & Disclaimer

The information contained in this book is not designed to replace or take the place of any form of medication or professional medical advice. The information in this book has been provided for educational and entertainment purposes only.

The information contained in this book has been compiled from sources deemed reliable, and it is accurate to the best of the Author's knowledge. However, the Author cannot guarantee its accuracy and validity so cannot be held liable for any errors or omissions. Changes are periodically made to this book. You must consult your doctor or get professional medical advice before using any of the suggested remedies, techniques, or information in this book.

Upon using the information contained in this book, you agree to hold harmless the Author from and against any damages, costs and expenses, including any legal fees, potentially resulting from the application of any of the information provided by this guide. This disclaimer applies to any damages or injury caused by the use and application, whether directly or indirectly, of any advice or information presented, whether for breach of contract, tort, negligence, personal injury, criminal intent, or under any other cause of action.

You agree to accept all the risks of using the information presented inside this book. You need to consult a professional medical practitioner in order to ensure you are both able & healthy enough to participate in this program.

Contents

Introduction 3

Chapter 1: Understanding Mistakes 4

Chapter 2: The Positivity of Making Mistakes 8

Chapter 3: The Fear of Failure 11

Chapter 4: Various Methods to Overcome Fear of Failure 17

Chapter 5: How to Learn from Mistakes 27

Conclusion: Learn to Forgive Yourself 32

Check Out Other Books 37

Introduction

Will you like to be successful in life? Would you like to have meaningful success in learning, developing, and making a significant contribution, where your life is full, counts for something, and makes a difference? If your answer is "YES," then you must learn to overcome mistakes and failures. There is no exception to that rule. That's what this book is all about—understanding the concepts of mistakes and failure and learning how to overcome them to achieve your full potential and become successful in life.

Failure is one of the most feared words in English. The very thought of failure is enough to stop most of the people in their tracks. It can cause the majority to simply pack up, turn around, and retreat without even trying. Success, on the other hand, is almost a mystical concept for most people. People want to be considered a success and will always sacrifice a great deal to achieve this goal.

Failure is often related to a lack of potential to succeed in the face of a particular task, but obvious failures can be a powerful way to learn and, ironically, provide the means for life's greatest breakthroughs and successes. Eventually, we will come to understand that what other people call failures are typically just temporary setbacks.

In this book, you will learn:

- Why failure is actually good for you

- Why you are afraid of failure and how you can overcome this fear

- How to get the most out of the mistakes you have made in life

- How to forgive yourself and move on with life when you failed or made a mistake

- And more!

If you have just encountered a major setback in life, and need some form of motivation to bounce back from failure, this might be the right book for you. So, let's learn together and move on with life! We will start off by understanding what is meant by "mistakes"

Chapter 1: Understanding Mistakes

What is a mistake?

A mistake is a goof, a slip-up. You did something wrong when you made a mistake. A mistake has a lot of uses, but they've all got to do with the wrong thing. A mistake in a math class would result in a wrong answer, but a mistake with a gun could kill someone. If you mix up two people, you're going to mistake one for the other.

Reasons why people make mistakes

Nobody is perfect. All humans are susceptible to errors. Stress, pressure, and poor concentration are a few factors that will affect our performance. Therefore, we are prone to errors as a result of our different biological, emotional, mental, and physical characteristics

Some are used to working without enough sleep or in a nosy environment, but when things aren't as they usually are, that's when they tend to make more mistakes. Stress, Mental strain, Short-term memory, and Wrong mindset are some of the factors that make a person more likely to make mistakes.

Stress, whether real or perceived, results in problems like making people panic, or inhibiting their ability to remember, think, or act. Stress also causes anguish, fear, memory lapses, or even make one unable to think rationally or execute physical tasks accurately. The consequences are equally adverse, regardless of whether the stress is at work or home.

Mental strain is another factor. As humans, we don't like to engage in a task for long hours because it requires a high level of attention, concentration, and effort. If you've ever been to a training session and you can't understand why you're so exhausted after a long day of training, that's the reason why. With mental strain, we begin to accept "okay" output or quality levels as anything else is too difficult.

Our short-term memory can only remember a limited number of things at a time, typically 5 to 8 things. Hence, this explains why we are sometimes "forgetful", which causes us to perform a task poorly by forgetting altogether. How many items do you need to remember at a point in time? How frequent do you forget to do something since you need to remember so many things?

Usually, we can only focus on a maximum of 3 things at one go. What we're going to focus on is the thing that we think is most important. If something else turns out to be more important than what we wanted to focus on, we're going to have a slip, lapse, or mistake. E.g. if we start thinking about getting a gift for our partner, that's going to take all our attention. As a result, we might forget when is his/her birthday and deliver the gift on the wrong date. Hence, the likelihood of error is higher if you have too many things to attend to.

A wrong mindset also increases the likelihood of mistakes occurring. Most individuals pay attention to the end goal, such as manufacturing 200 units daily. As a result, we work towards achieving the target and might overlook any issues that occur during the process. In the above example where the target is to manufacture 200 units daily, we might overlook the quality of raw materials used in the manufacturing process. It is therefore important to clarify what are the pitfalls to avoid and what must be done in the process.

It is hard to spot your own mistakes. Hence, self-checking is not a silver bullet in stopping mistakes.

A person cannot perform optimally if he is feeling tired. You will understand this best if you are a parent taking care of an infant or toddler, as you will realise that a lack of sleep makes you more likely to make mistakes.

Many people, despite knowing that they are not at an optimal level, still push themselves to perform tasks. Often, you see people coming to work even when they feel unwell. If you need to clear a huge backlog of work or any impairment, this also puts you at a "below optimal" level, which increases the likelihood of human error.

We need to know what leads to us making mistakes. This allows us to analyze them and think of ways to minimise them. Inadvertent errors can be divided into three categories.

1. Slips – do something incorrectly despite knowing what to do.
2. Lapses – forget to do something, or lose track of what you are doing in the middle of a task due to poor concentration.
3. Mistakes – do something wrong but believe what you did is correct because you misinterpreted or misapplied your knowledge.

Slips and lapses happen in familiar tasks that we can perform without thinking too much, e.g., driving. When we get distracted, even for a few seconds, this is where a slip or lapse tend to happen, and before we know it, 'whoops'. Noise or distractions around us makes it more likely to occur. We tend to slip when we return to a task after being interrupted by phone and e-mail. We could confuse two similar tasks, like keying in numbers on two spreadsheets and realising that we keyed in the numbers in the wrong spreadsheet. If a process involves many complicated steps, we might inadvertently miss a step or two. Or maybe we're good at high-level detail, but tend to slip at fine details.

All of us are vulnerable to slips and lapses due to poor concentration. Here are some examples:

- Fill the kettle but forget to switch it on
- Did not wear safety equipment before performing the task
- Key the wrong number on the spreadsheet

- Pick the wrong bolt because they look similar.
- Read a wrong dial or record data incorrectly
- Pick up the wrong job sheet

Training is not the answer for slips and lapses. So now the question is, what can we do to get rid of slips and lapses? The aviation sector is constantly working in these areas to continue to operate as a safe form of transportation. Some of the things they do include:

- Educate everyone about slips and lapses, so that people don't get shock when it happens – don't blame. Instead, think of how to prevent them or mitigate its repercussions when it happens.
- Include checklists in the process that will be reviewed by two people
- Make sure that all processes are easy, rational, and simple to follow;
- Start procedures by explaining issues and solving them
- Eliminate unnecessary interruptions. E.g. no calls;

The other unintentional human error is mistakes. Mistakes occur when someone thinks he is doing the right thing, but he is not. It is not doing the wrong thing on purpose but due to not understanding the situation.

Normally, this kind of error occurs when we're attending to a lot of things at one go. E.g. forgetting to attach a file for a sales proposal because we need to make ten other proposals at that point in time. Time pressure, as well as working on a lot of complicated things at the same time, also contributes to mistakes. As a result, something wrong will happen, and this is when mistakes are going to be made.

Examples of such mistakes entail:

- A bad judgment when overtaking
- Don't hear the alarm on the machine because you concentrate on other things.
- Not meeting the deadline because you have too much work to do

What increases the likelihood of us making mistakes?

- The environment in which we work - too hot, dim lighting, limited workspace, noise
- The type of work we do - huge workloads, dull and repetitious tasks, tasks that involves constant concentration, a lot of interruptions.
- Social issues – peer pressure, incorrect attitudes towards health and safety, different opinions on how to complete a task, fewer workers.
- Individual stressors – inadequate sleep, family issues, poor health
- Problems with equipment – incorrect or confusing instructions and procedures
- Organizational issues – failure to understand where errors can occur and to implement controls, such as training and monitoring

QUESTIONS
- What is a mistake?
- What are the various reasons people make mistakes?

Chapter 2: The Positivity of Making Mistakes

No matter how talented an individual thinks they are, it's not going to stop making mistakes. Throughout history, we as humans have made minor and major mistakes that change history as we know it. Even though most people see negatives in making mistakes, they're surprisingly positive along with making mistakes.

Then, the first thing is that everyone makes mistakes for different reasons and different ways, as we have already outlined on the previous page.

When you work at a station for a long time, there will be days when you're bored or tired of doing the same old thing. This leads you not to give your whole effort and attention to the task. Later, because of your careless attitude to your task, you make a careless mistake. For those who are less experienced, they are prone to mistakes in their work, especially because they haven't been used to performing the work. This leads to a lack of practice, wonders, and questions, and at last, to forget the steps in their work.

Now, the catch in making mistakes is that they could happen anywhere. Although they could happen anywhere, it's easier for them to get to some places than others.

Mistakes are part of being a human. Acknowledge your mistakes and most importantly, remember that some life lessons are only learned by making a mistake. Below is a positive side to making mistakes.

1. It makes you serve as a learning experience for others who are watching you:

    People tend to feel scared to mess up because they don't want to ever be judged. Well, you never know until you try and make a mistake that overcomes your fear. Not only do you overcome fear, but it can also serve as a learning experience for others and this can help them overcome their fear too. Hence, it is actually good to expose yourself to failures, as it can serve as a learning experience both for yourself, and anyone else watching you make the mistake.

2. It brings comedy and excitement to life in general:

    Never laugh at someone's mistake in making them feel bad, but take a sense of having a relatable mistake of your own that you did or still did. For your info, it's usually more respectful to laugh at the harmless mistake that someone has made than the one that is more serious or fatal. Also, the best circumstances mistakes can lead to laughter is when both you and the person making the mistake are laughing. Have you seen someone make a random but silly mistake in something like a sport or a dance? Then you laughed a little because it seems hilarious. Don't you think that's another positivity of making mistakes? There's a sense of laughter, a mixture of lessons all in one, from seeing mistakes in this life.

3. It gives you a lot more thought and allows you to be open-minded:

    When you made a mistake in an experiment or a math question, you become more determined to find out how to do it correctly. Mistakes push us to look longer and harder for the right solution to the success step. The more we try, the easier it will be for us to survive, and the same statement goes for making a mistake. Ultimately, you are walking on a more adventurous path to success when you make a mistake, and that might be better. You'll be more willing to hear someone else's advice (respectful advice) if they decide to tell you their experiences.

4. It makes your confidence to be kept in check:

    Many people seem super confident and tough until they make a mistake. Some people in life need a reality check that they're not at the top of the world. Especially those who love to point out other people's flaws when they have their flaws to look at. When those kinds of people make mistakes, they don't believe they're as cocky and loud as they were when they got it all right.

5. Mistakes are creating compassion and understanding:

    Man, when I tell you that mistakes give us a sense of care and understanding, it really does. Mistakes give us the heart to be more loving and to accept those who mess up because when people mess up, it gives us a reflection of all of us in action. We are all human beings; no one is ever perfect at all. We have moments when we feel like we're perfect, but unfortunately, those moments don't last. So just remember to cheer on when they shine like you want others to do for you.

6. Mistakes give you the experience you may need to grow:

    Mistakes come from experience, but so is a success. You can only succeed in doing something and experience the tenseness of acting. Trust me because I was there, but the mistakes could be better teachers than the school teachers. People tend to scold or criticise someone when they see the person making a mistake, but they never dare to actually do what the person does. Deep and important in my mind, it's better to learn from doing than any other way of life. Then, the only way you can make a mistake is by doing something more than talking or watching to gain the experience you need, which can change who you are forever in a good way.

7. You're going to be a leader in your own mysterious way:

   If you are being judged or insulted for making a mistake, ignore the judges and the haters. Usually, a person who likes to point out other people's errors do so because they are not strong enough to point out their own mistakes. When you mess things up and own it, it is a testament of your bravery, acceptance, action, and teaching all in one, all of which are traits of an effective leader. In life, we need mistakes to live and encourage others to live. Every person had to fail at something before they could officially succeed at something in their life at some point. We all need to look at someone else's mistake in order to learn and gain some sense of positivity. Also, someone needs to see your mistakes to make you feel the same good at the same time. In reality, no matter how experienced you are, how talented you are, you, me, and every living creature will make a mistake. This leads us to say that every single person and creature in this life is equal.

QUESTIONS

- Outline the various positive aspects of making mistakes

Chapter 3: The Fear of Failure

"If you try and fail

Congratulations

Most people don't even try"

What is Failure?

Failure can be defined as the total absence or lack of success. This is a fairly universal purpose definition. It allows us to personally define success so that we can know whether or not we have failed. The main problem here is that most of us are not great at defining success. This could make us think we are a failure when the reverse is actually true. Working and living this way does not recognise or value all the small achievements in our lives. It's time for a redefinition.

Why We Are Often Afraid of Failing

Below are the main reasons for fear of failure:

1. Perfectionism

    Adopting a perfection mindset is the main reason why one is afraid of failing. For individuals who adopt the perfection mindset, failing is very horrible and embarrassing to them, to the extent that they dare not try in the first place. Getting out of your comfort zone is terrifying.

    Things have never been perfect. Life is imperfect here. Life is all a series of mistakes and failures.

2. False Self-Confidence

    An individual with false self-confidence dares not take risk. They prefer the "safe way" of not trying anything new to avoid failure. People with true trust know they're not always going to succeed.

3. Unhealthy Organization Culture

    Most organizations today over-emphasize on perfection and does not accept any failure.

    Imagine the stress and terror of an organization like that. The persistent covering up the smallest imperfections or pushing the blame. Misleading, dishonesty, fabrication of information, and concealing issues—until the matter escalates to a level where it can no longer be hidden.

4. You think what happened in the past will happen in the future.

   It's wrong! Sometimes, you may not achieve success unless you've had a couple of failures. Life always changes. Nothing will ever remain the same, even if you desire it too.

How The Fear of Mistakes and Failure Holds You Back

Mistakes and failure are sometimes the best teachers. Without them, you would be clueless. Mistakes and failure are also inherent sources of wisdom that you gain at birth and continue to make throughout your life. How else would you know how to walk if you'd never fallen down and figure out how to pick yourself up again?

Below are various reasons why it is bad to avoid mistakes or failure:

1. Miss out on Valuable Opportunities

   If some people fail to find a complete answer because of the lure of some early success, many more fail because they insist on proving that what worked for them previously still works, even if it doesn't anymore.

   They steer away from any further creativity, afraid that this time they could perhaps fail, reducing the luster that they try to keep their names from the past triumph.

   Besides, they feel that the success of something new could maybe prove that the achievements they've made in the past haven't been so great after all. Why take the risk when you can hang on to your reputation by not doing anything?

   These individuals are so heavily immersed in their egos and past greatness that they chose to set aside the opportunity for potential glory rather than risk the chance of failure.

2. "Successful" people give up on trying and lose out

   Talent sometimes becomes a problem. People with past successes like to win and meet high standards. This can make them so scared of failure that they're ruining their lives. When a positive trait, like an achievement, becomes too powerful in someone's life, it's on the way to becoming a major obstacle.

   Accomplishment is an effective value for many successful people. They built their lives on it. They achieve everything they do: school, college, sports, the arts, hobbies, work. Every new accomplishment adds value to the power of their lives.

   Gradually, failure becomes inconceivable. Perhaps they have never failed in anything they have done, so they have no experience of getting over it. Failing is perceived as the greatest nightmare for them: a frightening horror that must be avoided at all costs.

The easiest way to avoid failure is to never take any risks, stick strictly to what you know you can do, safeguard yourself, work the longest hours, double and carefully inspect everything, and be the most observant and conservative person in the universe. This absolutely helps, even though it is not completely sustainable in life.

If persistent hard work, dedication, brutal work schedules, and harrying subordinates do not prevent the possibility of failure, you will use every other means possible to keep it away.

3. Loss of creativeness

   Everybody loves to be successful. The problem arises when the fear of failure hinders you from trying, nor understand the essence of trials and mistakes in discovering the most creative solution; if you dare not make mistakes, you will never see your creativity

4. You lose the experience.

   You need to experience what isn't working. This is how science experiments and research are conducted. When you apply this to your life, the results of the experience will stick. They're going to enter your subconscious and stay there. You can't learn if you don't make a mistake.

5. You can't reach the top without them.

   Mistakes and failures are building blocks, each laying the foundation for future success. As Mark Cuban said, "I learned a lot with every effort. With every mistake and failure, not only mine but those around me, I've learned what I can't do."

6. You will listen to the negative voices in your head.

   You're allowing negativity to live in your head. You can never achieve happiness if your life is governed by negative emotions.

   If you give "I can't, I'm afraid to fail" a negative attitude, say hello to a boring life.

7. You stagnate and underachieve.

   Nothing good can happen unless you're willing to make mistakes. Follow the bliss.

   Say good-bye to success if you're afraid to try new things and make mistakes!

8. You lose the opportunity to be strong.

   You'll never know how powerful you are unless you have a chance to bounce back from setbacks.

According to Bruce Lee, "Mistakes are always forgivable if you have the courage to admit them."

9. You lose the opportunity to be wiser.

    You won't realise how intelligent you are unless you made a mistake, get back up again and learn from it.

10. You become a quitter, not a winner.

    You are admitting defeat if you allow your mistakes to control you. Bill Gates said, "We didn't miss cell phones, but the way we went about it didn't allow us to take the lead. So, it's clearly a mistake." Nevertheless, he didn't let that setback impede him from being one of the richest people in the world through his other efforts.

11. If you don't learn from your mistakes, you will learn nothing.

    When things didn't work out, it doesn't mean that something good didn't come out of it. Amazing discoveries can happen because of mistakes.

12. You will become a negative role model.

    Bouncing back from setbacks is a real victory. Others are observing you, whether it's your child, your colleagues, or your subordinates (if you're a team leader). Would you like to be a good role model or a bad role model? It is not whether or not you made a mistake. What matters more is whether you're going to sink or swim. Successful leaders will swim after their mistakes. Michael Jordan was denounced when he made a bad draft call for the Bobcats, and he said, "I think we've grown out of it. I grew up on it, and hopefully, down the road, when you make a choice, you're trying to make a better choice."

13. You don't get to see the benefits of repetition.

    Practicing helps you build your skills. You must practice the task again and again if you want to be successful. Based on Malcolm Gladwell's "10,000 Hour Rule," grandeur is formed after repeating it for over ten thousand hours. The secret to mastery in a task is to carry out that particular task 20 hours a week for ten years.

14. No pain, no gain.

    After working out at the gym for hours, your body hurts, but you love it. Ironic, isn't it? This is because you feel satisfied for putting in all these efforts to improve yourself. You may even enjoy all the aching while you were exercising, although you didn't look very happy at that point in time.

15. You surrender to your fears.

    You're going to become frozen when you envision failure. You allow your fears to dominate your life and decide your future.

    Life without mistakes or failure is an incomplete life. Nothing is greater than reflecting on your experiences, how you overcame challenges, and what you learnt. The real failure is those who don't get up after a mistake or failure.

Why It Is Hard to Accept Failure

1. We focus on the outcomes and neglect the process

    Most people will ask "What do you do?" at the start of a conversation, rather than, "How would you describe yourself?" From the cradle to the grave, we look only at the outcomes, what we have achieved or intend to achieve, rather than what really matters in life – what we love and how we try to enjoy what we love and what comes out of it. Most education systems put emphasis on results, not the process of learning. And when we start work, it's no different. "How much are you earning?" "When is your next promotion?" It would be much better to ask, "What do you enjoy most about your work?" Or, "What do you feel is your strength?"

2. Our lives are too isolated

    Some of the news we get is obtained remotely, and when we receive news in this way, we unavoidably receive only a small part of the overall picture. For instance, when we watch the Olympics, we see the race, but not the months and years spent preparing for the race. When we watch a film, we see only successful shots, not those hundreds of cut shots. Yet, there is so much more to life than just finished products, as mentioned in the previous point. To maintain a realistic view of what success is all about, we need to meet more regularly with people we love and trust, share experiences, successes, and even failures to create the foundation for success. Failures are building blocks of resilience, internal strength, and self-confidence.

3. We have been raised to focus on success

    As a child, you have probably been praised more for your successes than for the effort you have made. However, whether or not you succeeded depended on several things that were not in your control – the timing of the race or the exam, who else took part, etc. However, how hard you tried, and whether you kept trying, was – and is – totally in your control. If we want to help our children cope with failure more adaptively, we need to praise them for their hard work, much more than for the grade they are awarded or the order in which they finish the race.

4. We're not selfish enough

    To succeed, you have to commit to practice and fail at something several times first. You have to love what you're doing for that level of perseverance. You have to listen to yourself (rather than what you think other people expect from you) so that you can gain the courage to try again after failing until you succeed

5. We believe that we can set the future

    We have so much trouble dealing with failure because of our misconception about the future. We assume that the future is manageable, that we can set a goal and then simply achieve it. If that is the case, life is not fun. A goal is more like a hypothesis that could be amended several times along the way. Would you like to become a doctor? If that guess is correct, you're going to love work enough to push through the setbacks, the late nights, and the letdowns. As you better understand your passion, you might realise that the reason why you aspire to become a doctor is because you love biology. Perhaps what you really want is to become a botanist or a zoologist. You may even realise that helping people unleash their greatest potential makes you feel fulfilled in life, so instead of becoming a physician, you may want to consider human performance or sports coaching. Failure teaches you something, and should be seen as an opportunity to learn.

QUESTIONS

- How do you define failure?
- List the various reasons why we are often afraid of failure
- What are the various ways the fear of failure holds you back?
- What are the various reasons why it is bad to avoid making mistakes?
- Why do you think it is difficult to accept failure?

Chapter 4: Various Methods to Overcome Fear of Failure

Fear is something that we all experience, especially when we set up a new undertaking. The fear of failing is probably the most prevalent and harmful fears that people are struggling with. However, remember that the first step of success is failure. A successful person like Michael Jordan (former professional National Basketball Association player) is open about his countless failures and how this has influenced his success. Just avoiding the feeling of fear is unlikely; nevertheless, you can take a close look at your fear of failure and then work with it to define your future success. Continue reading to learn how to overcome your fear and achieve your goals.

METHOD 1: REFRAME YOUR FAILURE

1. Recognize failure as a learning experience.

   Failure is a necessary part of the learning process when people master a skill or project. Learning requires exploration and creativity, and both of these approaches provide an opportunity to learn what doesn't work and what does. We can't explore the depths of what knowledge has to offer until we try it out. Embarking failure as a learning experience allows you to see it as a gift, not a punishment or a sign of weakness.

   Don't forget that many people went through the same situation. Take for example Myshkin Ingawale, an inventor from India known for inventing a bloodless anemia test to turn smartphones into mobile medical labs. It took him 32 iterations before he finally developed a prototype of his technology that worked. He could have given up and described himself as a failure after any of those roadblocks, but he continued to focus on learning from his mistakes and applying them to the future, and today his invention has reduced maternal death rates in rural India by fifty percent.

2. Re-assess your approach.

   Often, when the result doesn't match our expectations, we're tempted to attempt a failure. It is an "all or nothing" mindset, where you perceive everything as either a yes or no, rather than to examine it in a nuanced way. However, if we consider our results to be more or less effective, with the aim of improving them, we can always make positive changes.

   - Studies show that successful people do not usually encounter fewer or more setbacks than people who are not. The key is exactly how you interpret the failure. Setbacks does not prove that it's impossible for you to succeed.

- It takes time and hard work to achieve your idealized results. Failure is a step towards success. You should continue this process and not let the thought of failure stop you
- Don't run away from failure. Instead, accept the fact that failure will only help you produce better results.
- Remember that you can't control or predict it all. View unexpected variations or fluctuations as they are: external elements beyond your control. Only account for what's in your control.
- Make sure your goals are realistic and feasible. You can make use of the "SMART" method (Specific, Measurable, Attainable, Realistic, and Timely) when setting the goals.

Specific: Simple, precise, and unambiguous

Measurable: With clear criteria that evaluate the progress towards achieving the goal

Achievable: Attainable and not impossible to accomplish

Realistic: Within the scope, reasonable and relevant to the purpose of your life.

Timely: With a clearly specified timeline, including the start date and the target date. The aim is to create urgency.

3. Take things slow

Running into new ventures unprepared makes matters worse. You're going to have to manage your fear of failure slowly.

- Try to find the smallest steps you can take to achieve the goals that you feel comfortable with.
- Think of any long-term or large-scale goals in terms of those small steps you know you can take.

4. Be kind to yourself.

Don't make fun of your fears; they're there for a reason. Work with your fears, treat yourself with sympathy and understanding. The more you learn why you have these fears and what causes them, the better you can work with them.

- Write down your fears. Be as detailed as possible and have the courage to figure out what you're afraid of and why.
- Accept that your fears are part of you. Doing so helps you regain control of them.

5. Take some notes.

   Learning from the past is crucial to building a better future for yourself. Keep track of what worked, what didn't, and why. Plan any future actions in line with what you have learned from past actions.

   - Improving your future plans by keeping track of what works and what doesn't work will help to ease the fear of failure.
   - Learn how to value failure. Failure is as informative and valuable as success.
   - Experience failure will allow you to learn from what didn't work and help you avoid that setback in future attempts. You will likely still face challenges, roadblocks, and setbacks, but you will be better equipped to overcome them with the knowledge you have gained.

METHOD 2: WORK WITH THE FEAR OF FAILURE

1. Look deeper into your fear of failure.

   Often, fear of failure is only a general understanding of what we are truly afraid of. If this fear of failure is examined, it may be discovered that it is underpinned by other fears. These specific fears can be addressed and worked with once they have been identified.

   - Fear of failure is often only a broad level of understanding of what the problem is.
   - We may be afraid to fail, but failure is often linked to other ideas, such as self-esteem, self-image, and shame.
   - Examples of more specific fears may include fear of losing security from a risky investment or of being exposed to humiliation by your peers.

2. Avoid personalizing and over-generalizing failures.

   It can be easy to see something that you interpret as a failure and to extend the lack of success to yourself. You may also take a single instance of failure and apply it to your entire life and self. You might think, "I'm a loser" or "I'm worthless" because your efforts don't have the results you're hoping for. While this is common, it's not helpful, and it's not true either.

   Take a look at the script in your head about this event. We often allow our thoughts to slip into predictable, unhelpful scripts. For example, if you're working on an invention and the 17th attempt has just been bombed, you might experience this script: "Yeah, I'm never going to get that right. I'm a failure." The facts of the situation are that this attempt has not worked. The facts say nothing about you as a person or about the possibility of success in the future. Separate the facts of your script.

3. Stop the perfection mindset.

It is a misconception that perfectionism is the same as healthy ambition or excellence. On the contrary, perfectionism can lead to failure. Perfectionists are often obsessed with fears of failure. They often categorize anything that does not meet their unreasonably high standards as "failure." This can lead to things like procrastination because you are so concerned that your work is imperfect that you can never finish it. Set up healthy, ambitious standards for yourself, and acknowledge that sometimes your work is not going to meet them.

Perfectionism may also make you more likely to develop mental health conditions such as depression and eating disorders.

4. Stay positive.

Sometimes, it is actually simple to focus on past failures and let them prevent you from succeeding in the future. Instead of focusing solely on how badly things seem to have gone, focus on what went well and what was learned.

- Even if your main goal has not been successful, you can still be successful if you learn from the experience.
- Focusing only on negative aspects will make the situation appear to be completely negative.
- By focusing on success and positive aspects, you will learn what works and be better prepared for the future.

5. Keep learning.

If you're afraid of failing with a new task or you're worried about failing with a familiar one, you can keep your skills up to date to help with that. Practicing your skills allows you to witness how competent you really are, which increases your self-confidence. Recognize what you are doing well, as well as the areas in which you can develop further.

- Strengthen your existing skills. Always keep up to date with any new best practices that might be used in this skill set.
- Learn about new skills. By learning new skills, you will enhance your skill set and be better prepared for a wider range of situations that may arise as you pursue your goals.

6. Take action.

The only real failure is the one that happens when you never try. Taking the first step is generally the most difficult one; however, it is also the most important one. It's natural to feel scared and uncomfortable when you try something new. You can take a few steps to help you deal with this discomfort.

- Permit yourself to feel uncomfortable with that. Everyone will feel uncomfortable to take on more challenges at some point in life, even famous billionaires. Recognize that it is natural to feel like this, and don't be tempted to suppress it. Rather, let yourself experience the feeling even if you feel scared.
- Remember to break down your larger targets into smaller ones. Having these smaller stages that you know you can achieve will make the larger goal less intimidating.
- Moving forward will provide you with new information and allow you to adjust your course of action towards success.

7. Subject yourself to failing.

This means intentionally and actively going through the experience of failure. The goal of this practice is to help you realise that failure is not as frightening as you might think it is. This is a technique known as exposure therapy and can be used to reduce the effects of fear in your life. Doing this will make you more comfortable in handling fear or discomfort. Also, this method will reinforce the principle that you will eventually succeed after failing.

- Think of a new hobby or activity that you're not qualified to do. Practice that hobby or activity and anticipate yourself to fail in the process. Most importantly, always remember that these failures will only increase your future success.
- For example, start playing a new instrument. Failures to correctly play the instrument along the way will be common. These failures will give you a lot of opportunities to get comfortable with failure. They will also show you that failure is neither total nor debilitating. Just because you're going to fail the first hundred times you try to play the Moonlight Sonata doesn't mean you're never going to get it right.
- When you buy something, consider negotiating for a rebate. Your intention is to fail, to reframe failure, and to nullify the limiting effects that fear may have on your actions.

METHOD 3: OVERCOME THE PANIC CAUSED BY FEAR

1. Realize that you're panicking.

Like other fears, the fear of failure may trigger physiological reactions similar to panic attacks or anxiety attacks. To stop this type of panic attack, the first thing you need to do is to realize the symptoms at the onset of a panic attack. Look for a few of the following symptoms:

- Faster heart rate or erratic rhythm of the heart.
- Breathing difficulties or stiffness of the throat.
- Tingling, trembling, or perspiring.
- Feeling light-headed, sleepy, or as if you're about to pass out.

2. Take a deep breath.

When you experience a panic attack, you will breathe quickly and shallowly which will only maintain the state of panic. To regain control of your breathing, breathe in deeply and slowly to help bring your breath back to a normal rhythm.

- Breathe through your nose slowly, for five seconds. Use your diaphragm, not your chest, to breathe. Your stomach is supposed to rise with your breath, not your chest.
- Exhale at the same slow pace, through your nose again. You should completely release all the air in your lungs, counting to 5 while doing so.
- Repeat this breathing cycle until you begin to feel calm.

3. Relax your muscles.

Your body is likely to experience tension when you have a panic attack, which only amplifies to the feeling of anxiety. Work to release tension in your muscles by tensioning, holding, and releasing those muscles.

- You can tense and release all the muscles in your body at once for a quick and complete body relaxation technique.
- For greater relaxation, start by tensioning the muscles in your legs, holding them for a few seconds, and then release it. Move your body, then repeat the same process for your arms, back, chest, face, neck, shoulders, and stomach.

METHOD 4: OVERCOME NEGATIVE THOUGHTS

1. Try S.T.O.P.P.

S.T.O.P.P. (Stop, Take, Observe, Pull, Proceed) can help you avoid responding to situations of immediate fear. When you encounter the fear of failure, practice the following:

- **S**top what you're going to do. Whatever you do, stop and take a step back from the situation. Give yourself some time to think about it before you react.
- **T**ake a deep breath, please. Clean yourself up through a series of deep breaths. Doing so allows oxygen to flow to your brain normally, so that you can think more clearly.

- **O**bserve what's going on. Just ask yourself a few questions. What's going on in your mind? What do you feel? What's the "script" in your head right now? Are you looking at the facts? Do you give more weight to opinions? What do you focus on?
- **P**ull back for perspective. Put yourself in the perspective of an unprejudiced witness. How would the person view the situation? How else can this situation be approached? How big is this situation in the grand scheme of things—is it going to matter six days or six months from now?
- **P**roceed according to your principles. Go ahead with what you know and have determined. Practice what is most in line with your values and objectives.

2. Confront negative self-talk.

The worst critics is often ourselves. You may find that it is always your inner critic that is grumbling how woefully inadequate you are. Do you often hear your inner critics saying "I am bad at this", "I'm never going to get that right", or "I shouldn't even bother trying that"? Once you realise that such thoughts are forming, confront them as they are not helpful and untrue.

- Think about how you would advise a friend. Imagine that it's a friend or a loved one in your situation. Maybe your best friend is afraid to leave her day job to pursue her dream of becoming a musician. What would you say to her? Can you imagine her failure at once, or can you find ways to support her? Give yourself the same kind of compassion and the same belief that you would show a loved one.
- Think about whether you're generalizing. Are you taking a specific example and generalizing it to your entire experience? For example, if your science project has not worked, do you extend that failure to every aspect of your life and say something like, "I'm a failure?"

3. Don't catastrophize.

Catastrophizing means you assume that the worst thing that could possibly happen is going to happen. When you catastrophize, your fears will hinder you from thinking rationally, causing you to jump to conclusions and think that the worst is happening. To stop yourself from catastrophizing, slow down and ask for proof of your assumptions.

- For instance, you may be worried that if you change your college major to a subject that you really want to study but find challenging, you will fail. From there, your thoughts could spiral into a catastrophe: "If I fail this major, I'm going to flunk out of college. I'm never going to find a job. I'm going to have to live in my parents' basement for the rest of my life. I'm

never going to be able to date or marry or have children." Obviously, this is an extreme case, but it's an example of how fear can wildly send your thoughts to the left field.
- Try to put your thoughts into perspective. For instance, you may be concerned that you're going to fail if you change your course of study in University. More importantly, you should consider the possible worst-case scenario, and how likely is that? In this case, the worst thing that's going to happen is that you're not good at organic chemistry (or whatever the subject attracts you), and you're going to miss a few courses. It is not a catastrophe. You can do many things to overcome these failures, like spending more of your free time to study, or talking to professors.
- The more likely situation is that you will find your new subject difficult at first, but you will learn and grow and finish college, happy to pursue your passion.

4. Recognize that you are usually the worst critic of your own.

The fear of failure may stem from the belief that others are scrutinizing every move you make. You may feel like a little slip-up is going to be noticed and spread around. However, the fact is that most people are so engaged in their own issues and worry that they don't have the time or effort to scrutinize every little thing you do.

- Look for evidence that goes against your assumptions. For example, you might be worried about going to parties because you're afraid you might say something silly or make a joke about the bombs. This fear of failure may keep you from enjoying social interactions with others. However, you can overcome this fear by learning from any similar experience other people might have had in the past.
- For instance, you might think about whether any of your friends or anyone you know has ever made a social faux pas. It's pretty much guaranteed that you can think of someone who had a social slip-up. Did their mistake result in them being shunned or everyone seeing them as a failure? It's probably not.
- Whenever you feel afraid that you will fail and be criticised by others, remember: "Nobody is perfect. So, I shall allow myself to make a mistake. Just because I made a mistake doesn't mean I am a failure."
- When you receive hurtful comments from over-critical people, recognize that the problem is with them, not with you.

Flowchart

1. Reframe your failure
- Recognise failure as a learning experience
- Re-assess your approach
- Take things slow
- Be kind to yourself
- Take some notes

2. Work with the fear of failure
- Look deeper into your fear of failure
- Avoid personalizing and over-generalizing failures
- Reject perfectionism
- Stay positive
- Keep learning
- Take action
- Expose yourself to failure

3. Overcome the panic caused by fear
- Realise that you are paniking
- Take a deep breath
- Relax your muscles

4. Overcome negative thoughts
- **S**top, **T**ake, **O**bserve, **P**ull, Proceed
- Challenge negative self-talk
- Avoid catastrophizing
- Recognize that you are usually the worst critic of your own

QUESTIONS

- List the various methods we can overcome the fear of failure

Chapter 5: How to Learn from Mistakes

Have you ever made a mistake that has had severe repercussions in your life? What about a small mistake that ended up innocuous but still makes you embarrassed to think about it? Everyone has regrets, and everyone has made mistakes. From time to time, these mistakes might return to haunt you. But mistakes might not always be a negative thing. In fact, when you learn from your mistakes, you can experience great personal growth.

Below are several ways we can learn from our mistakes.

1. Be aware of your mistake

    This may sound obvious, but it's actually one of the hardest parts of it. Why? Why? Because we've got a hard time dealing with our imperfections.

    It's common to feel defensive or guilty when we make mistakes. We lash out, look for others to blame, or minimize the impact. We're really making it about how we're not "bad."

    That's why you've got to kill the idea that the mistakes are bad. When you make a mistake, practice saying, "Okay, okay. That was a mistake on my part. It might have been avoided, but it wasn't. I need to deal with it now and figure out how to do better in the future."

2. Determine the cause of the mistake

    Once more, you might find that feeling to blame others for the mistakes. But this isn't helpful. You're simply looking for things that you can change when you determine the cause.

    Your friend may have kept you talking late on the phone, so you didn't get enough sleep. But you have chosen to talk on the phone.

    Your boss may have sent a vague email. But you were not asking for clarification.

    You might have thought you'd read the email carefully. Perhaps the fault lies with your boss. But even here, you're not powerless. You can adjust how you interact with your boss in the future to prevent miscommunication from happening again.

3. Ask yourself some tough questions

   What's in the way of you achieving your goal? Anything that slows you down or prevents you from making progress toward that goal is an obstacle.

   They can be physical challenges, mental blocks, emotional drawbacks, or family impediments.

   You admitted that you were wrong and isolated the pieces under your control. Now there are some tough questions you need to address:
   - What are the consequences of this mistake for my immediate future?
   - How did the mistake negatively affect those around me?
   - Are there any ways to correct the mistake?
   - If not, can I compensate for the damage?
   - Am I the only one to blame for what happened?
   - If other people are also at fault, how can I reach them so that it doesn't happen again?

4. Listen to feedback

   The responses you get differ depending on the circumstance. It could come from your manager, workmates, relatives, friends, or even strangers.

   Try not to see criticisms as people attacking you or drilling on your flaws. Rather, use criticisms as a chance to improve. Take the observations of the people into account.

   Sometimes they'll have suggestions on how to avoid repeating the mistake in the future. Sometimes they're just going to tell you the outcome of your mistakes. All in all, these feedbacks point out vital information on how you can deal with the situation.

5. Come up with a plan

   The plan you use will also vary depending on the complexity of the situation. Your plan should, as a general rule, address:
   - How to fix the error or mitigate its consequences to the best of your ability
   - How to interact with those harmed by the mistake
   - How to resolve and eradicate the root source of the mistake
   - How to assume accountability for people in your life
   - How to remain accountable

6. Create powerful routines

    Strong routines are vital to the organization and essential to performance-based error. If you're still making the same mistake with your software or phone script, you need to practice it. Consistent routine is the key to build a new habit.

    Routines also facilitate your error troubleshooting process. Identifying the cause is easier, and creating a plan with practice.

7. Teach other people your lessons

    When you learn from your mistakes, they don't always have to be your own. You can learn from other people's mistakes. Others can learn from you, too.

    You might have come up with a great system to read emails without missing information. You might have a mental trick to remember a complicated coding issue. The solutions you create can help others. Try to teach them if you see them making the same mistakes you used to make.

    Think of the experts you respect and the things they teach. How many of their tricks do you think they've learned through their own trial and error?

8. Expand your thinking

    As we get older, we start to "settle" our thoughts. It's getting harder to challenge our preconceptions and learn new things.

    That's why you need to make a productive effort to expand your thinking. Never think of yourself as someone who has grown up. Instead, think of yourself as someone who has an ever-changing potential. Tell yourself that you'll know something you didn't know about today tomorrow. Then, at the end of the day, find something you know that you didn't know yesterday.

Flowchart

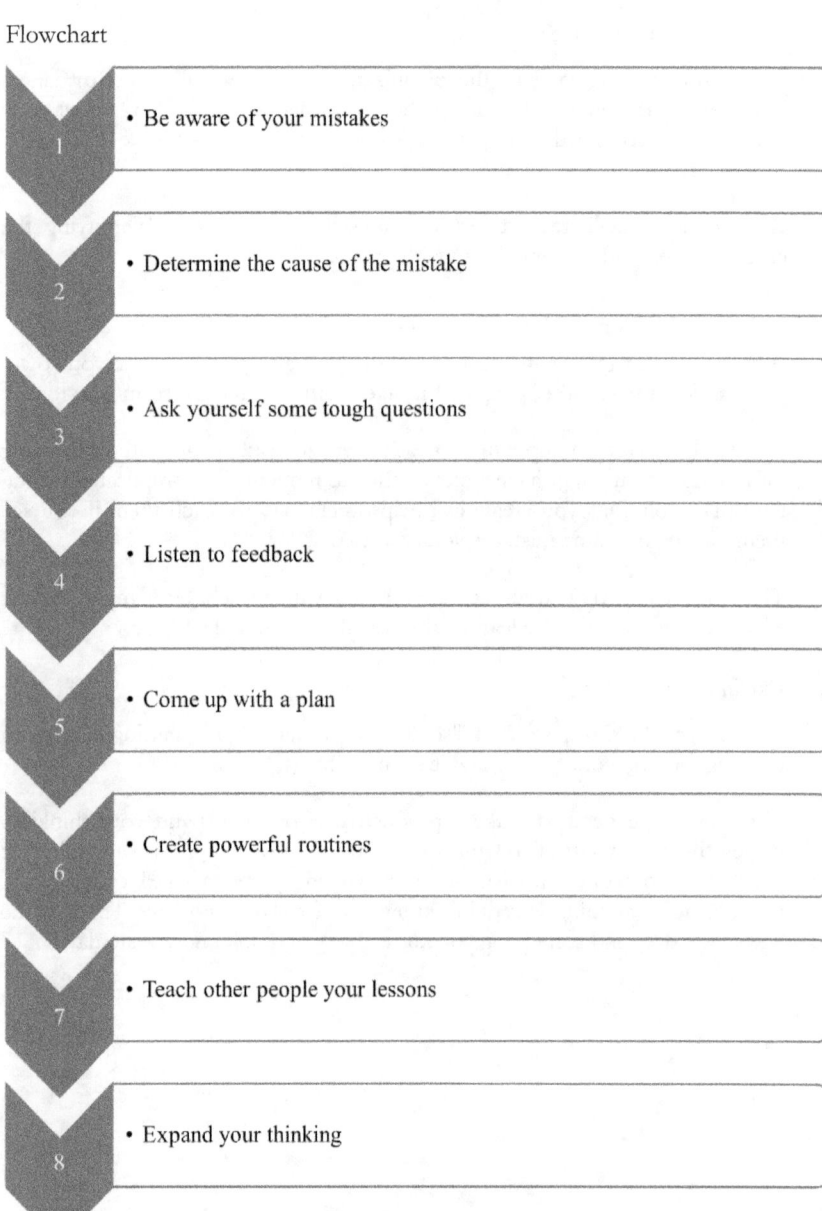

1. Be aware of your mistakes
2. Determine the cause of the mistake
3. Ask yourself some tough questions
4. Listen to feedback
5. Come up with a plan
6. Create powerful routines
7. Teach other people your lessons
8. Expand your thinking

QUESTIONS

- List the various ways we can learn from our mistakes

Conclusion: Learn to Forgive Yourself

After a failure, some persons feel self-hatred. This set of people often equate failing to a failure person. As a result, they fall into the downward spiral of negative self-criticism, which hinders their ability to handle failure constructively and rise from disappointment. If you suffer from this problem, you need to learn how to turn self-criticism into self-compassion before you move on.

The question is, what can you do to put an end to self-criticism and be more compassionate to yourself instead? Read on to find out how

1. Imagine that your friend is dealing with failure and you want to help him

    Unless you are the worst friend in the world, I suppose that if a friend of yours experienced failure, you would console him, not criticise, right? So, why do we lend kindness to others but don't extend it to ourselves?

    It's hard to feel self-empathy when you're mad at yourself. It's easier to feel empathetic towards someone else because then you look at the situation as a bystander, free from the negative emotions that cloud your judgment. Why don't you also look at yourself from that perspective?

    Imagine that you are writing a letter to your best friend, who happens to be an exact copy of you. What would you say to this person to help them overcome their feelings of inadequacy and self-hatred that arose out of failure? How would you convey the compassion that you feel towards them? What would you write to remind this person that every person fails and that it doesn't mean that they're inferior? How are you going to communicate that you understand the situation in which they found themselves and tell them that you care?

    When you finish writing your letter, get it out of sight and forget about it. A few days later, open the letter, read it, and allow its compassionate tones sink into you. Reading the letter will help you be more understanding and compassionate to yourself.

2. Reframe your critical self-talk

    Your inner critic could be a great ally if his criticisms were constructive. However, the reality is that our inner critics tend to be negative and make destructive remarks like "you are useless", instead of something constructive like "you did not get it done correctly because you were distracted by other tasks."

Why don't you turn your internal criticisms into something useful? The first step is to become aware of when your negative self-talk is present and how it speaks to you. Then, as a person watching a critic instead of being a critic, you can hear a message, dissect it, and turn it into something more useful.

I know it sounds a bit out there, so let's plunge into some more detailed instances: You were dieting. One day, you were handling a traumatic issue and as a result, you treated yourself to unhealthy snacks as a way to console yourself. You might hear your critical self-talk making remarks such as, "You screwed it up again. You had to mess it all up and comfort yourself with food. You are such a weak-willed loser!"

If you're looking for the underlying message, "You're an emotional eater," you can extract something useful from this self-criticism. But before you do that, show yourself some compassion. More importantly, recognise the challenges you face.

You were going through hardships, and need to have a connection with yourself. Food always make you feel better when you need some form of consolation, so you give up your diet to make yourself feel better. Clearly, you need to lighten your mood when you are feeling blue, otherwise, you wouldn't have been able to deal with this painful problem.

When you don't feel so remorseful or at the minimum, understand why you made that choice, reflect on the negative outcome of your actions. You may have solved the problem, but you did it at the expense of your diet, and eventually, your health.

What else can you do to get in touch with yourself other than eating? Could you try to connect with yourself by meditating, reading a book, walking, listening to your favorite music, watching your favorite TV show, exercising, or doing anything else that makes you feel okay but is not self-destructive?

If it has to be eating, can there be at least something less caloric and healthier to eat? If you can't, can you at least combine it with some exercise to reduce its negative effects on your well-being?

Also, try looking at the words of your inner critic from a different perspective. If you say, "You're lazy," you can admit, yes, sometimes you don't feel like doing things, and that may pose a problem, but at the same time, it's helpful because you're just investing your time and energy in something you find worthwhile.

If it says, "You can never focus on one thing at a time," you can agree that sometimes you need to focus more, but at the same time, your restlessness means that you have a lot of energy and curiosity that you can use to help you achieve your goal.

Examining self-criticism from another point-of-view helps you avoid thinking in black and white terms. Your weaknesses may cause problems, but they can also help, so why hate yourself for them?

3. Nurture yourself

    Failure often leads to discouragement, which then turns into a strong need to comfort oneself. Pampering yourself when you feel bad will help you gain access to a more positive state of mind, which will help you overcome your self-critical voice. If you beat yourself up with never-ending self-criticism, you're only going to drive yourself deeper into the abyss of guilt. As a result, it will take you even longer to bounce back.

    According to scientific research, if you exhibit self-compassion after you fail to meet your goals, you will increase your mental resilience. Self-kindness is also helpful in dealing with procrastination and increases positivity.

Flowchart

1. Imagine that you're helping a friend deal with failure

- Look at yourself from a 3rd person perspective
- Encourage yourself, not criticise
- Write a letter to yourself, reminding yourself that everyone fails, and failure is not inferior. Read the letter a few days later

2. Reframe your critical self-talk

- Do not say you are useless, loser, failure or anything bad about yourself
- Criticise your **approach** or **why** you failed, but it must not be anything negative about **yourself**

3. Nurture yourself

- Pamper yourself
- Do not self-criticise anymore

QUESTIONS

- What are the various ways we can forgive ourselves for our mistakes or failure?

Check Out Other Books

Go here to check out other related books that might interest you:

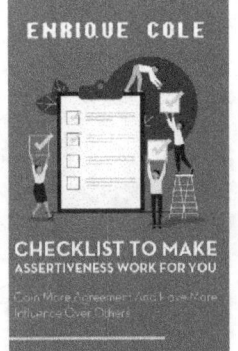

Checklist to Make Assertiveness Work for You
https://www.amazon.com/dp/B08T7G2JXQ

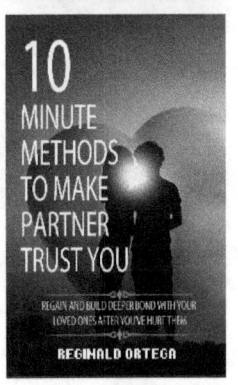

10-Minute Methods to Make Partner Trust You
https://www.amazon.com/dp/B08Z8C297V

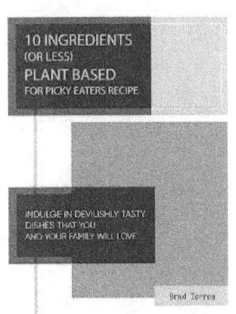

10 Ingredients (Or Less) Plant Based for Picky Eaters Recipe
https://www.amazon.com/dp/B09KQPJS6Q

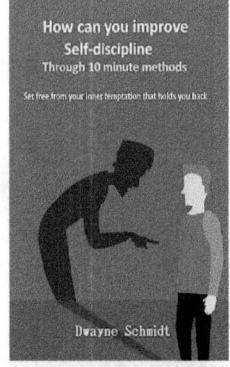

How Can You Improve Self-discipline Through 10 Minute Method
https://www.amazon.com/dp/B09KQQTS2W

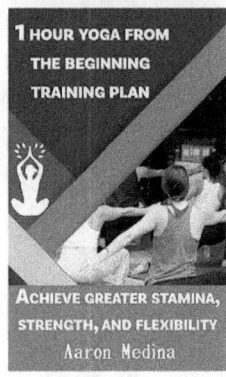

1 Hour Yoga from The Beginning Training Plan
https://www.amazon.com/dp/B09KQPKLNF

www.ingramcontent.com/pod-product-compliance
Lightning Source LLC
Chambersburg PA
CBHW071221240526
45470CB00018B/2196